A Journey
Histor

Uncovering the Mysteries of an Ancient Practice

Copyright © 2023 by Deepa Norris.

All rights reserved. No part of this book may be reproduced or transmitted in any form or by any means, electronic or mechanical, including photocopying, recording, or any other information storage and retrieval system, without permission in writing from the publisher.

This book was created with the assistance of Artificial Intelligence technology. While every effort has been made to ensure the accuracy of the information contained herein, the author and publisher cannot be held responsible for any errors or omissions or any consequences arising from the use of the information in this book.

The contents of this book are for entertainment purposes only and should not be considered as professional advice. Readers should consult with a qualified professional before making any decisions based on the information provided in this book. The author and publisher disclaim any liability for any damages or losses, whether direct or indirect, that may arise from the use of this book.

Introduction: What is Yoga? 6

The Origins of Yoga: Ancient India 8

The Vedas and Early Yogic Philosophy 10

The Upanishads and the Emergence of Yoga as a Practice 13

The Yoga Sutras of Patanjali 15

Hatha Yoga: The Physical Branch of Yoga 17

The Nath Yogis and the Development of Hatha Yoga 19

The Importance of Breath: Pranayama 21

The Five Sheaths of the Body: Koshas 23

The Chakra System and the Science of Energy 26

The Divine Feminine: Shakti and Kundalini Yoga 29

Tantra: Beyond Hatha Yoga 32

The Bhagavad Gita and the Role of Karma Yoga 34

Jnana Yoga: The Yoga of Knowledge 36

Bhakti Yoga: The Yoga of Devotion 38

Yoga in the Medieval Period: The Bhakti Movement 40

Yoga and the Mughal Empire 42

The British Raj and the Modernization of Yoga 44

Swami Vivekananda and the Introduction of Yoga to the West 46

Theosophy and the Influence of Eastern Philosophy on Western Thought 48

The Yoga Renaissance: The 1960s and 70s 50

The Beatles and Maharishi Mahesh Yogi 52

B.K.S. Iyengar and the Development of Iyengar Yoga 54

Pattabhi Jois and the Ashtanga Vinyasa Yoga System 56

The Evolution of Modern Yoga: Vinyasa and Power Yoga 58

The Rise of Yoga in America: Yoga Journal and Yoga Alliance 60

Yoga and the Wellness Industry 62

Yoga and the Internet: Yoga in the Digital Age 64

Yoga and the Internet: Yoga in the Digital Age 66

Yoga and Pop Culture: Yoga in Film and TV 68

Yoga and Celebrity Culture 70

Yoga in India Today: The Role of the Government 72

Yoga in the West Today: Trends and Developments 74

Yoga and Science: The Benefits of Yoga 77

Yoga and Social Justice: The Intersection of Yoga and Activism 80

Conclusion: The Future of Yoga 82

Introduction: What is Yoga?

Yoga is an ancient practice that originated in India over 5,000 years ago. It is a discipline that combines physical, mental, and spiritual practices designed to enhance overall health and well-being. Yoga is often thought of as a series of poses, but in reality, it is much more than that. It is a way of life that encompasses the entire being and seeks to create balance and harmony between the body, mind, and spirit.

The word "yoga" comes from the Sanskrit word "yuj," which means to yoke or unite. This reflects the goal of yoga, which is to unite the individual with the divine or the universe. According to yogic philosophy, the individual is seen as a microcosm of the universe, and the goal of yoga is to bring the individual into harmony with the greater cosmic forces.

Yoga is often associated with Hinduism, but it is not a religion in itself. It is a spiritual practice that can be practiced by anyone, regardless of their religious beliefs. The practice of yoga has evolved over time, and there are now many different styles and approaches to yoga. However, all styles of yoga share the same underlying philosophy and principles.

One of the main components of yoga is the physical practice, known as asana. Asanas are the various poses that are held during a yoga practice. These poses are designed to stretch and strengthen the body, improve flexibility and balance, and promote overall physical health. In addition to the physical practice, yoga also includes pranayama, or breathing techniques, which help to calm the mind and increase focus.

Another important aspect of yoga is meditation. Meditation is a practice that involves focusing the mind on a particular object, thought, or activity in order to achieve a state of mental clarity and calmness. The goal of meditation is to quiet the mind and reduce mental chatter, allowing for a greater sense of inner peace and harmony.

Yoga also includes ethical and moral principles, known as the yamas and niyamas. These principles provide guidance for living a virtuous and fulfilling life. The yamas include non-violence, truthfulness, non-stealing, celibacy or moderation, and non-possessiveness. The niyamas include cleanliness, contentment, self-discipline, self-study, and surrender to a higher power.

In addition to its physical and spiritual benefits, yoga has been shown to have numerous health benefits. Studies have shown that yoga can help to reduce stress and anxiety, lower blood pressure, improve heart health, and alleviate symptoms of depression and anxiety. Yoga has also been shown to improve flexibility, balance, and coordination, as well as enhance overall physical performance.

Yoga has become increasingly popular in recent years, with millions of people practicing yoga around the world. While there are many different styles and approaches to yoga, all styles share the same underlying philosophy and principles. Whether you are looking to improve your physical health, reduce stress and anxiety, or deepen your spiritual practice, yoga offers a powerful and transformative path towards greater health and well-being.

The Origins of Yoga: Ancient India

The origins of yoga can be traced back to ancient India, where it was first developed over 5,000 years ago. The exact origins of yoga are unclear, but it is believed to have emerged as a spiritual practice among the ancient Vedic civilization of India.

The earliest evidence of yoga comes from the ancient texts known as the Vedas, which were written between 1500 and 500 BCE. The Vedas are a collection of hymns and rituals that were used by the ancient Vedic civilization to connect with the divine. The Vedas contain references to a variety of spiritual practices, including meditation, breath control, and ritual sacrifice, which are considered to be precursors to modern yoga.

The Upanishads, a collection of texts written between 800 and 400 BCE, further developed the spiritual practices of the Vedas and introduced the concept of inner knowledge, or jnana. The Upanishads also introduced the idea of karma, or the law of cause and effect, which became an important part of yogic philosophy.

The early yogis, or ascetics, were known as rishis, and they lived in the forests and mountains of India, dedicating their lives to the pursuit of spiritual knowledge and enlightenment. These yogis developed a variety of spiritual practices, including meditation, breath control, and physical postures, which are now known as asanas.

One of the most important texts in the development of yoga is the Yoga Sutras of Patanjali, which was written around

200 BCE. The Yoga Sutras outlines the eight limbs of yoga, which include ethical principles, physical practices, breath control, meditation, and contemplation. The Yoga Sutras also introduced the concept of samadhi, or a state of spiritual consciousness, which is considered to be the ultimate goal of yoga.

Hatha yoga, the physical branch of yoga, emerged during the medieval period in India, around the 11th century CE. The Nath yogis, a group of ascetics who practiced yoga in the forests of India, developed the practice of hatha yoga, which focused on physical postures and breath control techniques. The Nath yogis believed that the physical body was the vehicle for spiritual transformation and that by purifying the body through yoga, one could achieve spiritual liberation.

The practice of yoga continued to evolve over time, with new styles and approaches emerging throughout India. In the 19th and early 20th centuries, yoga began to gain popularity in the West, with figures like Swami Vivekananda and Paramahansa Yogananda introducing yoga to Western audiences.

Today, yoga is practiced by millions of people around the world and has become a popular form of exercise, stress relief, and spiritual practice. While the origins of yoga may be ancient, its message of spiritual transformation and inner peace remains relevant and inspiring to people of all backgrounds and beliefs.

The Vedas and Early Yogic Philosophy

The Vedas are a collection of ancient texts that were written in India between 1500 and 500 BCE. These texts are considered to be the oldest and most sacred scriptures of Hinduism and are an important source of information about the early history of yoga.

The Vedas consist of four main texts: the Rigveda, the Yajurveda, the Samaveda, and the Atharvaveda. These texts contain hymns, prayers, and rituals that were used by the ancient Vedic civilization to connect with the divine. The Vedas also contain references to a variety of spiritual practices, including meditation, breath control, and ritual sacrifice, which are considered to be precursors to modern yoga.

The Upanishads, which were written between 800 and 400 BCE, are a collection of texts that further developed the spiritual practices of the Vedas and introduced the concept of inner knowledge, or jnana. The Upanishads also introduced the idea of karma, or the law of cause and effect, which became an important part of yogic philosophy.

The early yogis, or ascetics, were known as rishis, and they lived in the forests and mountains of India, dedicating their lives to the pursuit of spiritual knowledge and enlightenment. These yogis developed a variety of spiritual practices, including meditation, breath control, and physical postures, which are now known as asanas.

The Rigveda contains references to a variety of spiritual practices, including meditation, breath control, and ritual sacrifice. One hymn in the Rigveda describes the practice of pranayama, or breath control, and another hymn describes the practice of dhyana, or meditation.

The Yajurveda contains instructions for a variety of rituals, including fire ceremonies and offerings to the gods. The Yajurveda also contains references to the practice of yoga, including descriptions of the eight limbs of yoga and the practice of meditation.

The Samaveda contains hymns that were used in ritual chanting and singing. These hymns are considered to be a form of meditation and were used to connect with the divine.

The Atharvaveda contains a variety of spells and incantations, as well as references to the practice of yoga. One hymn in the Atharvaveda describes the practice of pranayama, while another describes the practice of meditation.

The early yogic philosophy that emerged from the Vedas and Upanishads emphasized the importance of spiritual knowledge and the pursuit of inner peace and harmony. The yogis believed that the body was the vehicle for spiritual transformation and that by purifying the body and mind through yoga, one could achieve spiritual liberation.

The early yogis also believed in the concept of maya, or the illusion of reality. They believed that the material world was an illusion and that the true nature of reality was spiritual. This concept is still a fundamental part of yogic philosophy today.

In conclusion, the Vedas and early yogic philosophy laid the foundation for the development of yoga as a spiritual practice. The ancient texts contained within the Vedas and Upanishads provide valuable insights into the early history of yoga and the spiritual practices that emerged from it. Today, yoga remains a powerful tool for achieving physical, mental, and spiritual well-being, and its roots can be traced back to the ancient wisdom of the Vedas and Upanishads.

The Upanishads and the Emergence of Yoga as a Practice

The Upanishads are a collection of ancient texts that were written in India between 800 and 400 BCE. These texts are considered to be some of the most important and influential scriptures of Hinduism and are an important source of information about the history and development of yoga.

The Upanishads build upon the teachings of the Vedas and introduce the concept of inner knowledge, or jnana. They also introduce the idea of karma, or the law of cause and effect, which became an important part of yogic philosophy. The Upanishads contain many references to yoga and provide valuable insights into the early development of yoga as a spiritual practice.

The Upanishads introduce the concept of atman, or the individual soul, and brahman, or the universal soul. They suggest that the individual soul is a microcosm of the universal soul and that the goal of yoga is to realize the ultimate unity of these two souls.

The Upanishads also introduce the idea of maya, or the illusion of reality. They suggest that the material world is an illusion and that the true nature of reality is spiritual. This concept is still a fundamental part of yogic philosophy today.

One of the most important Upanishads for the development of yoga is the Katha Upanishad. This text describes the practice of yoga and the path to spiritual enlightenment. It emphasizes the importance of self-control and the need to overcome the senses in order to achieve spiritual liberation.

The Upanishads also introduce the concept of meditation as a means of achieving spiritual enlightenment. They describe various techniques for meditation, including the use of mantras, or sacred words, and the practice of breath control, or pranayama.

The Upanishads also contain references to the practice of asanas, or physical postures. These postures were originally used as a means of preparing the body for meditation, but they eventually became an important part of hatha yoga, the physical branch of yoga.

The Upanishads provide valuable insights into the early development of yoga as a spiritual practice. They emphasize the importance of inner knowledge, self-control, and spiritual liberation. They introduce the concept of maya, or the illusion of reality, and suggest that the true nature of reality is spiritual. They also introduce the practice of meditation and the use of physical postures as a means of achieving spiritual enlightenment.

In conclusion, the Upanishads played a crucial role in the emergence of yoga as a spiritual practice. They laid the foundation for the development of yogic philosophy and introduced key concepts and practices that are still a fundamental part of yoga today. The Upanishads provide valuable insights into the early history of yoga and the spiritual practices that emerged from it.

The Yoga Sutras of Patanjali

The Yoga Sutras of Patanjali is a text that was written in India around 200 BCE. It is considered to be one of the most important and influential texts in the history of yoga, and it provides a comprehensive guide to the practice of yoga and the attainment of spiritual liberation.

The Yoga Sutras consist of 196 aphorisms, or short verses, that are organized into four chapters. The first chapter focuses on the nature of yoga and its benefits, while the second chapter describes the practice of yoga and the eight limbs of yoga. The third chapter describes the various psychic powers that can be achieved through the practice of yoga, while the fourth and final chapter describes the ultimate goal of yoga, which is spiritual liberation.

The first chapter of the Yoga Sutras describes the nature of yoga and its benefits. It suggests that yoga is a means of calming the mind and achieving inner peace and happiness. It also suggests that the practice of yoga can lead to the attainment of supernatural powers, such as telepathy and clairvoyance.

The second chapter of the Yoga Sutras describes the practice of yoga and the eight limbs of yoga. The eight limbs include yama, or ethical principles; niyama, or self-discipline; asana, or physical postures; pranayama, or breath control; pratyahara, or sense withdrawal; dharana, or concentration; dhyana, or meditation; and samadhi, or spiritual absorption.

The third chapter of the Yoga Sutras describes the various psychic powers that can be achieved through the practice of yoga. These powers, known as siddhis, include the ability to levitate, the ability to become invisible, and the ability to control the elements.

The fourth and final chapter of the Yoga Sutras describes the ultimate goal of yoga, which is spiritual liberation. It suggests that through the practice of yoga, one can achieve a state of samadhi, or spiritual absorption, in which the individual soul merges with the universal soul. This state of spiritual liberation is known as kaivalya.

The Yoga Sutras of Patanjali provide a comprehensive guide to the practice of yoga and the attainment of spiritual liberation. They describe the nature of yoga and its benefits, as well as the practice of yoga and the eight limbs of yoga. They also describe the various psychic powers that can be achieved through the practice of yoga and the ultimate goal of yoga, which is spiritual liberation.

The Yoga Sutras have had a profound impact on the development of yoga as a spiritual practice. They have influenced the development of many different styles of yoga, including Hatha yoga, Ashtanga yoga, and Iyengar yoga. The principles outlined in the Yoga Sutras continue to be a fundamental part of yoga philosophy and practice today.

Hatha Yoga: The Physical Branch of Yoga

Hatha yoga is the physical branch of yoga that focuses on physical postures, breath control, and meditation. Hatha yoga is derived from the ancient practice of yoga, and it emerged during the medieval period in India, around the 11th century CE.

The term "hatha" is derived from the Sanskrit words "ha" and "tha," which mean "sun" and "moon" respectively. Hatha yoga is often described as a balancing of the sun and moon energies within the body, with the sun representing active, masculine energy, and the moon representing passive, feminine energy.

The practice of hatha yoga is designed to purify the body and mind, preparing them for the pursuit of spiritual knowledge and enlightenment. The physical postures, known as asanas, are designed to improve flexibility, strength, and balance, while also helping to release tension and promote relaxation.

There are many different styles of hatha yoga, each with their own unique approach to the practice. Some popular styles of hatha yoga include Iyengar yoga, which focuses on precise alignment and the use of props, and Ashtanga yoga, which is a fast-paced, flowing style that emphasizes strength and endurance.

One of the most important texts for the practice of hatha yoga is the Hatha Yoga Pradipika. This text, written in the 15th century CE, provides a comprehensive guide to the practice of hatha yoga, including instructions for physical postures, breath control, and meditation.

The physical postures, or asanas, are a central part of hatha yoga. They are designed to improve flexibility, strength, and balance, while also promoting relaxation and reducing stress. Some popular asanas in hatha yoga include downward-facing dog, child's pose, and warrior pose.

Breath control, or pranayama, is another important component of hatha yoga. Pranayama techniques involve controlling the breath in order to improve energy flow and promote relaxation. Some popular pranayama techniques in hatha yoga include alternate nostril breathing and ujjayi breathing.

Meditation is also a key component of hatha yoga. Meditation techniques involve focusing the mind on a specific object, such as the breath or a mantra, in order to calm the mind and promote inner peace. Some popular meditation techniques in hatha yoga include mindfulness meditation and mantra meditation.

In conclusion, hatha yoga is the physical branch of yoga that focuses on physical postures, breath control, and meditation. The practice of hatha yoga is designed to purify the body and mind, preparing them for the pursuit of spiritual knowledge and enlightenment. Hatha yoga is a popular form of exercise and stress relief, and it has been shown to have a wide range of physical and mental health benefits. Whether you are new to yoga or an experienced practitioner, hatha yoga is a powerful tool for improving your overall health and well-being.

The Nath Yogis and the Development of Hatha Yoga

The Nath Yogis were a group of yogis who emerged in India during the 10th century CE. They were followers of the Nath tradition, which combined elements of yoga, Tantra, and Shaivism. The Nath Yogis played a key role in the development of hatha yoga, the physical branch of yoga.

The Nath Yogis believed that the body was the vehicle for spiritual transformation, and they developed a variety of physical and breathing techniques to purify the body and mind. They believed that by purifying the body and mind, one could achieve spiritual liberation.

One of the most important figures in the development of hatha yoga was Matsyendranath, a legendary Nath Yogi who is believed to have lived during the 10th century CE. Matsyendranath is credited with developing many of the physical postures, or asanas, that are now a central part of hatha yoga.

Another important figure in the development of hatha yoga was Gorakshanath, another Nath Yogi who lived in the 11th century CE. Gorakshanath is credited with developing many of the breathing techniques, or pranayama, that are now a central part of hatha yoga.

The Nath Yogis believed in the importance of physical postures, or asanas, as a means of preparing the body for meditation. They developed a variety of asanas that were designed to improve flexibility, strength, and balance, while also promoting relaxation and reducing stress.

They also emphasized the importance of breath control, or pranayama, as a means of purifying the body and mind. They developed a variety of pranayama techniques that were designed to improve energy flow and promote relaxation.

The Nath Yogis believed in the concept of kundalini, or the energy that lies at the base of the spine. They believed that through the practice of hatha yoga, one could awaken this energy and channel it upwards towards spiritual liberation.

Nath Yogis were also known for their use of mudras, or hand gestures, and bandhas, or energy locks, as a means of controlling the flow of energy in the body.

The Nath Yogis were influential in the development of hatha yoga, and their teachings continue to be a fundamental part of yoga philosophy and practice today. The physical postures, breath control techniques, and spiritual concepts that were developed by the Nath Yogis are now a central part of hatha yoga and are practiced by millions of people around the world.

In conclusion, the Nath Yogis played a key role in the development of hatha yoga, the physical branch of yoga. They developed a variety of physical and breathing techniques that were designed to purify the body and mind, and they emphasized the importance of preparing the body for meditation. The teachings of the Nath Yogis continue to be a fundamental part of yoga philosophy and practice today, and they have had a profound impact on the development of yoga as a spiritual practice.

The Importance of Breath: Pranayama

Pranayama is the yogic practice of controlling the breath, and it is considered to be one of the most important aspects of yoga. Pranayama is a Sanskrit term that means "life force extension," and it is believed to have a wide range of physical and mental health benefits.

The practice of pranayama involves controlling the breath through various techniques, such as deep breathing, alternate nostril breathing, and ujjayi breathing. These techniques are designed to improve energy flow, calm the mind, and promote relaxation.

Pranayama is a central component of hatha yoga, the physical branch of yoga, and it is also a key aspect of other forms of yoga, such as Ashtanga yoga and Kundalini yoga.

The benefits of pranayama are numerous. Studies have shown that pranayama can help to reduce stress and anxiety, lower blood pressure, improve lung function, and boost immune function. Pranayama is also believed to improve concentration, increase energy levels, and promote better sleep.

One of the most popular pranayama techniques is ujjayi breathing, also known as ocean breath. This technique involves breathing through the nose and creating a sound in the back of the throat, similar to the sound of ocean waves. Ujjayi breathing is believed to calm the mind and promote relaxation.

Another popular pranayama technique is alternate nostril breathing, also known as nadi shodhana. This technique involves breathing through one nostril at a time, alternating between the left and right nostrils. Nadi shodhana is believed to balance the flow of energy in the body and promote a sense of calm and relaxation.

The practice of pranayama can be done at any time, but it is often done in conjunction with physical postures, or asanas. The combination of asanas and pranayama is believed to be particularly effective for promoting physical and mental health.

In conclusion, pranayama is the yogic practice of controlling the breath, and it is considered to be one of the most important aspects of yoga. Pranayama techniques are designed to improve energy flow, calm the mind, and promote relaxation, and they have been shown to have a wide range of physical and mental health benefits. The practice of pranayama is a fundamental part of yoga philosophy and practice, and it is a powerful tool for improving overall health and well-being.

The Five Sheaths of the Body: Koshas

In yoga philosophy, the body is believed to be composed of five sheaths, or layers, known as koshas. Each kosha represents a different aspect of the body, from the physical to the spiritual, and each sheath is said to be progressively more subtle than the one before it.

The five koshas are:

1. Annamaya Kosha: The Physical Sheath

The annamaya kosha is the physical sheath of the body, and it represents the physical body and its functions. This sheath is made up of the muscles, bones, organs, and other physical components of the body.

2. Pranamaya Kosha: The Breath Sheath

The pranamaya kosha is the breath sheath of the body, and it represents the body's energy or life force. This sheath is made up of the breath, or prana, and it is associated with the respiratory system and the chakras, or energy centers, of the body.

3. Manomaya Kosha: The Mental Sheath

The manomaya kosha is the mental sheath of the body, and it represents the mind and emotions. This sheath is associated with the nervous system and the brain, and it includes the thoughts, emotions, and perceptions of the individual.

4. Vijnanamaya Kosha: The Wisdom Sheath

The vijnanamaya kosha is the wisdom sheath of the body, and it represents the individual's higher consciousness and intuition. This sheath is associated with the intellect and the ability to discern truth from falsehood.

5. Anandamaya Kosha: The Bliss Sheath

The anandamaya kosha is the bliss sheath of the body, and it represents the individual's true nature, which is pure consciousness and bliss. This sheath is associated with the spiritual heart and the ability to experience oneness with the universe.

The concept of the koshas is important in yoga philosophy because it emphasizes the interconnectedness of the body, mind, and spirit. By understanding the koshas, practitioners of yoga can work to balance and harmonize these different aspects of themselves in order to achieve a state of physical, mental, and spiritual well-being.

One of the ways that practitioners can work with the koshas is through the practice of yoga nidra, a form of guided meditation that involves systematically moving through the koshas in order to reach a state of deep relaxation and inner awareness. In yoga nidra, the practitioner moves through each of the koshas, from the physical to the spiritual, in order to access deeper levels of consciousness and awareness.

In conclusion, the five koshas represent the different aspects of the body, from the physical to the spiritual. Understanding the koshas is important in yoga philosophy because it emphasizes the interconnectedness of the body, mind, and spirit. By working with the koshas, practitioners of yoga can achieve a state of physical, mental, and spiritual well-being, and they can access deeper levels of consciousness and awareness. The practice of yoga nidra is one way to work with the koshas in order to achieve these states of consciousness and awareness.

The Chakra System and the Science of Energy

The chakra system is a key aspect of yoga philosophy, and it is believed to be an important part of the body's energy system. The chakras are energy centers located along the spine, and they are associated with different aspects of the body, mind, and spirit.

There are seven main chakras in the body, each of which is associated with a different color, sound, and element. The seven chakras are:

1. Muladhara Chakra: The Root Chakra

The muladhara chakra is located at the base of the spine, and it is associated with the color red and the element of earth. This chakra is associated with the physical body, survival, and grounding.

2. Svadhisthana Chakra: The Sacral Chakra

The svadhisthana chakra is located in the lower abdomen, and it is associated with the color orange and the element of water. This chakra is associated with creativity, sexuality, and emotional balance.

3. Manipura Chakra: The Solar Plexus Chakra

The manipura chakra is located in the upper abdomen, and it is associated with the color yellow and the element of fire. This chakra is associated with personal power, confidence, and self-esteem.

4. Anahata Chakra: The Heart Chakra

The anahata chakra is located at the center of the chest, and it is associated with the color green and the element of air. This chakra is associated with love, compassion, and forgiveness.

5. Vishuddha Chakra: The Throat Chakra

The vishuddha chakra is located at the throat, and it is associated with the color blue and the element of ether. This chakra is associated with communication, self-expression, and creativity.

6. Ajna Chakra: The Third Eye Chakra

The ajna chakra is located between the eyebrows, and it is associated with the color indigo and the element of light. This chakra is associated with intuition, wisdom, and insight.

7. Sahasrara Chakra: The Crown Chakra

The sahasrara chakra is located at the top of the head, and it is associated with the color violet and the element of thought. This chakra is associated with spiritual awakening, enlightenment, and unity with the divine.

The chakras are believed to be connected by a subtle energy system known as nadis, which are channels through which prana, or life force, flows. The practice of yoga, including physical postures, breath control, and meditation, is designed to balance and harmonize the chakras and nadis, in order to promote physical, mental, and spiritual well-being.

While the chakra system is a key aspect of yoga philosophy, it is also a subject of scientific study. Modern science has shown that the body's energy system, including the chakras and nadis, is intimately connected with the nervous system, endocrine system, and immune system. Studies have shown that the practice of yoga can have a wide range of physical and mental health benefits, including reducing stress and anxiety, improving lung function, and boosting immune function.

In conclusion, the chakra system is a key aspect of yoga philosophy, and it is believed to be an important part of the body's energy system. The chakras are energy centers located along the spine, and they are associated with different aspects of the body, mind, and spirit. The practice of yoga is designed to balance and harmonize the chakras and nadis, in order to promote physical, mental, and spiritual well-being. While the chakra system is a subject of spiritual study, it is also a subject of scientific study, and there is growing evidence to suggest that the practice of yoga can have a wide range of physical and mental health benefits. As modern science continues to explore the connections between the body's energy system and its various physiological and psychological functions, the chakra system is likely to play an increasingly important role in our understanding of human health and well-being. By integrating the ancient wisdom of yoga with modern scientific knowledge, we may be able to unlock new insights into the nature of the human body, mind, and spirit, and discover new ways to promote health, happiness, and spiritual growth.

The Divine Feminine: Shakti and Kundalini Yoga

In yoga philosophy, the divine feminine is represented by the goddess Shakti, who is considered to be the creative energy of the universe. Shakti is often depicted as a powerful and beautiful goddess, and she is associated with a wide range of qualities, including creativity, fertility, wisdom, and strength.

Shakti is also associated with the concept of kundalini, which is a powerful form of energy that lies dormant at the base of the spine. Kundalini energy is often described as a coiled serpent, waiting to be awakened and unleashed. When kundalini energy is awakened, it is said to rise up through the chakras, purifying and energizing the body and mind.

The practice of kundalini yoga is designed to awaken and harness this powerful energy, in order to achieve greater physical, mental, and spiritual well-being. Kundalini yoga involves a wide range of practices, including physical postures, breath control, meditation, and chanting, all of which are designed to activate and direct the flow of kundalini energy.

One of the key aspects of kundalini yoga is the use of mantra, or sacred sound. Mantras are used to focus the mind and direct the flow of energy, and they are believed to have a powerful effect on the body and mind. Chanting mantras is a central part of kundalini yoga, and it is believed to be a powerful tool for achieving spiritual growth and transformation.

Another important aspect of kundalini yoga is the use of specific physical postures, known as kriyas. Kriyas are sequences of movements and breath work that are designed to stimulate and energize the body, and to awaken the flow of kundalini energy. Kriyas may be practiced in conjunction with specific mantras, and they are believed to have a wide range of physical and mental health benefits.

The practice of kundalini yoga is closely linked to the concept of tantra, which is a spiritual tradition that emphasizes the unity of the individual self with the divine. Tantric practices often involve the use of sexual energy as a means of achieving spiritual transformation, and they are closely associated with the worship of Shakti as the divine feminine.

The concept of the divine feminine is an important aspect of yoga philosophy, and it is a powerful reminder of the importance of balance and harmony in all aspects of life. By honoring and connecting with the divine feminine within ourselves and within the universe, we can achieve greater physical, mental, and spiritual well-being, and tap into the infinite creative potential of the universe.

In conclusion, the concept of the divine feminine is an important aspect of yoga philosophy, and it is represented by the goddess Shakti and the powerful energy of kundalini. The practice of kundalini yoga is designed to awaken and harness this powerful energy, in order to achieve greater physical, mental, and spiritual well-being. The use of mantra, physical postures, and other techniques are all designed to activate and direct the flow of kundalini energy, and to help practitioners achieve spiritual growth and transformation. The concept of the divine feminine is a powerful reminder of the importance of balance and harmony in all aspects of life, and it serves as a guide for those seeking to tap into the infinite creative potential of the universe.

Tantra: Beyond Hatha Yoga

While hatha yoga is perhaps the best-known form of yoga in the West, there is another branch of yoga that is closely related to hatha yoga but is often misunderstood or misrepresented. This branch of yoga is known as tantra, and it has a rich and complex history that goes back thousands of years.

At its core, tantra is a spiritual tradition that emphasizes the unity of the individual self with the divine. Tantra teaches that the universe is a manifestation of the divine, and that everything in the universe is ultimately connected. The goal of tantra is to achieve a state of oneness with the divine, and to experience the infinite joy and bliss that comes from this state of consciousness.

Tantra is often associated with sexual practices, and while sexuality is certainly an important aspect of tantra, it is only one aspect of a much larger spiritual tradition. Tantra encompasses a wide range of practices, including meditation, yoga, mantra, ritual, and more. These practices are all designed to help the practitioner achieve a state of spiritual awakening, and to connect with the divine in a deep and profound way.

One of the key teachings of tantra is the concept of shakti, or the divine feminine energy that is present in all things. Shakti is often depicted as a goddess, and she is associated with qualities such as creativity, fertility, wisdom, and strength. In tantra, the worship of shakti is seen as a path to spiritual awakening, and it is often associated with the practice of kundalini yoga.

Kundalini yoga is a form of yoga that is closely related to tantra, and it is designed to awaken and harness the energy of kundalini, which is said to lie dormant at the base of the spine. When kundalini energy is awakened, it rises up through the chakras, purifying and energizing the body and mind. The practice of kundalini yoga is often accompanied by specific mantras, physical postures, and other techniques that are designed to activate and direct the flow of kundalini energy.

Another important aspect of tantra is the use of ritual, which is seen as a powerful tool for connecting with the divine. Tantric rituals may involve the use of specific symbols, such as yantras or mandalas, as well as the use of specific mantras and physical postures. These rituals are designed to help the practitioner achieve a state of heightened awareness and spiritual connection.

In conclusion, tantra is a spiritual tradition that emphasizes the unity of the individual self with the divine. Tantra encompasses a wide range of practices, including meditation, yoga, mantra, ritual, and more. The concept of shakti, or the divine feminine energy, is an important aspect of tantra, and it is often associated with the practice of kundalini yoga. While tantra is sometimes misunderstood or misrepresented in the West, it is a rich and complex tradition that has much to offer to those seeking spiritual growth and awakening.

The Bhagavad Gita and the Role of Karma Yoga

The Bhagavad Gita is one of the most important texts in yoga philosophy, and it has been a source of inspiration and guidance for yogis and spiritual seekers for thousands of years. The Bhagavad Gita is a dialogue between the warrior prince Arjuna and his charioteer, who is actually the god Krishna in disguise. The text is set on a battlefield, and it explores the themes of duty, morality, and spiritual growth.

One of the key teachings of the Bhagavad Gita is the concept of karma yoga, which is the yoga of action. Karma yoga is based on the idea that every action we take has consequences, and that we should strive to act in a way that is in alignment with our true nature and our highest ideals. In the Bhagavad Gita, Krishna teaches Arjuna that he must act according to his duty as a warrior, but that he should do so without attachment to the results of his actions. This is the essence of karma yoga.

Karma yoga is not about avoiding action or renouncing the world, but rather about acting in a way that is in harmony with our true nature and our highest ideals. Karma yoga involves selfless action, and it is based on the idea that we should act without attachment to the results of our actions. When we act in this way, we are able to transcend our ego and connect with the divine, and we are able to achieve a state of inner peace and spiritual fulfillment.

The practice of karma yoga involves a number of key principles, including selflessness, detachment, and surrender. Selflessness involves putting the needs of others before our own, and acting in a way that is in service to others. Detachment involves letting go of our attachment to the results of our actions, and recognizing that the outcome is ultimately beyond our control. Surrender involves letting go of our ego and connecting with the divine, and recognizing that we are part of a larger cosmic plan.

The teachings of the Bhagavad Gita and karma yoga have been a source of inspiration for countless yogis and spiritual seekers over the centuries. The message of selfless action, detachment, and surrender is as relevant today as it was thousands of years ago, and it is a powerful reminder of the importance of living in alignment with our highest ideals.

In conclusion, the Bhagavad Gita is a powerful text in yoga philosophy, and it teaches us about the importance of karma yoga, the yoga of action. Karma yoga involves acting in a selfless and detached way, and it is based on the idea that we should act in accordance with our true nature and our highest ideals. By practicing karma yoga, we are able to transcend our ego and connect with the divine, and we are able to achieve a state of inner peace and spiritual fulfillment. The teachings of the Bhagavad Gita and karma yoga have been a source of inspiration for countless yogis and spiritual seekers over the centuries, and they continue to be a powerful guide for those seeking spiritual growth and enlightenment.

Jnana Yoga: The Yoga of Knowledge

Jnana yoga is one of the four main paths of yoga, and it is the yoga of knowledge. Jnana yoga is based on the idea that the ultimate goal of human life is to achieve spiritual liberation, and that this liberation can be achieved through the acquisition of knowledge and wisdom.

In jnana yoga, the practitioner seeks to understand the true nature of the self, the world, and the divine. This understanding is not based on belief or faith, but rather on direct experience and realization. The goal of jnana yoga is to overcome ignorance and delusion, and to achieve a state of spiritual awakening and liberation.

The practice of jnana yoga involves a number of key principles, including self-inquiry, discrimination, and detachment. Self-inquiry involves asking the question "Who am I?" and seeking to understand the true nature of the self. Discrimination involves discerning between the real and the unreal, and recognizing that the world of appearances is ultimately illusory. Detachment involves letting go of attachment to the world and the ego, and recognizing that the true nature of the self is beyond all forms and identities.

Jnana yoga is often associated with the study of scriptures and philosophical texts, such as the Upanishads and the Bhagavad Gita. These texts are seen as a source of knowledge and wisdom, and they are studied and reflected upon in order to gain a deeper understanding of the nature of the self and the world.

The practice of jnana yoga is not limited to intellectual study and contemplation, however. It also involves the cultivation of certain qualities and attitudes, such as humility, openness, and receptivity. These qualities are essential for gaining a deeper understanding of the self and the world, and for overcoming the ego and the limitations of the mind.

Jnana yoga is a path that requires dedication, discipline, and a deep commitment to spiritual growth and self-realization. It is not a path for everyone, but for those who are drawn to it, it can be a powerful tool for achieving spiritual liberation and enlightenment.

In conclusion, jnana yoga is the yoga of knowledge, and it is based on the idea that spiritual liberation can be achieved through the acquisition of knowledge and wisdom. The practice of jnana yoga involves self-inquiry, discrimination, and detachment, as well as the study of scriptures and the cultivation of certain qualities and attitudes. Jnana yoga is a path that requires dedication, discipline, and a deep commitment to spiritual growth and self-realization. For those who are drawn to it, jnana yoga can be a powerful tool for achieving spiritual liberation and enlightenment.

Bhakti Yoga: The Yoga of Devotion

Bhakti yoga is one of the four main paths of yoga, and it is the yoga of devotion. Bhakti yoga is based on the idea that the ultimate goal of human life is to experience the divine love and devotion, and to develop a deep and personal relationship with the divine.

In bhakti yoga, the practitioner seeks to cultivate devotion and love for the divine through various practices, such as chanting, prayer, and the worship of deities. The goal of bhakti yoga is not to achieve spiritual liberation or enlightenment, but rather to experience the joy and bliss that come from a deep and personal relationship with the divine.

The practice of bhakti yoga involves a number of key principles, including surrender, devotion, and love. Surrender involves letting go of the ego and the illusion of control, and recognizing that the divine is the ultimate source of all power and wisdom. Devotion involves cultivating a deep and heartfelt love for the divine, and recognizing the divine in all beings and all things. Love involves experiencing the divine love and compassion, and sharing that love with others.

Bhakti yoga is often associated with the worship of deities, such as Krishna, Shiva, or the Divine Mother. The worship of these deities involves the use of specific mantras, prayers, and rituals, and it is seen as a way of connecting with the divine in a personal and meaningful way. The worship of deities is not seen as idolatry, but rather as a way of accessing the divine qualities and energies that these deities represent.

The practice of bhakti yoga is not limited to the worship of deities, however. It can also involve the cultivation of devotion through other practices, such as chanting, meditation, and selfless service. The goal of all these practices is to cultivate a deep and personal relationship with the divine, and to experience the joy and bliss that come from this relationship.

Bhakti yoga is a path that is accessible to anyone, regardless of their background or beliefs. It is a path that emphasizes the power of love and devotion, and it is a reminder that the ultimate goal of human life is not achievement or success, but rather the experience of divine love and compassion.

In conclusion, bhakti yoga is the yoga of devotion, and it is based on the idea that the ultimate goal of human life is to experience the divine love and devotion, and to develop a deep and personal relationship with the divine. The practice of bhakti yoga involves surrender, devotion, and love, and it can involve the worship of deities, chanting, meditation, and selfless service. Bhakti yoga is a path that is accessible to anyone, and it is a powerful reminder of the power of love and devotion to transform our lives and our relationship with the world.

Yoga in the Medieval Period: The Bhakti Movement

The medieval period in India saw the emergence of the Bhakti movement, a movement that emphasized devotion to a personal god or goddess. The Bhakti movement had a profound influence on yoga, and it played a key role in shaping the practice and philosophy of yoga as we know it today.

The Bhakti movement emerged in the 6th century CE, and it was a response to the rigid caste system and the dominance of the Brahmin priests in Indian society. The Bhakti movement emphasized the idea of divine love and devotion, and it encouraged people to worship a personal god or goddess in a way that was meaningful and accessible to them.

The Bhakti movement had a profound impact on yoga, and it helped to shift the focus of yoga from asceticism and self-denial to devotion and love. The Bhakti movement emphasized the importance of love and devotion in the practice of yoga, and it helped to popularize practices such as chanting, singing, and dancing as a way of connecting with the divine.

One of the key figures in the Bhakti movement was the poet-saints known as the Alvars and the Nayanars. These poets wrote devotional songs and hymns that were sung in temples and homes throughout India. Their poetry expressed a deep and heartfelt love for the divine, and it helped to popularize the idea of devotion and love as a central aspect of yoga practice.

The Bhakti movement also had an impact on the practice of hatha yoga, the physical branch of yoga. The Bhakti movement encouraged the use of physical postures, such as the asanas, as a way of expressing devotion and love for the divine. The physical practice of yoga was seen as a way of purifying the body and preparing it for the experience of divine love and devotion.

The Bhakti movement had a lasting impact on yoga, and it helped to shape the practice and philosophy of yoga as we know it today. The emphasis on love and devotion in the Bhakti movement helped to shift the focus of yoga from asceticism and self-denial to a more inclusive and accessible practice that emphasized the importance of the heart and emotions in the spiritual journey.

In conclusion, the Bhakti movement was a key development in the medieval period in India, and it had a profound impact on the practice and philosophy of yoga. The movement emphasized the importance of devotion and love in the practice of yoga, and it helped to popularize practices such as chanting, singing, and dancing as a way of connecting with the divine. The Bhakti movement also had an impact on the physical practice of yoga, and it helped to shift the focus of yoga from asceticism and self-denial to a more inclusive and accessible practice that emphasized the importance of the heart and emotions in the spiritual journey.

Yoga and the Mughal Empire

The Mughal Empire was a Muslim dynasty that ruled over large parts of India from the 16th to the 19th century. The Mughal emperors were known for their tolerance and patronage of the arts, including yoga and meditation.

During the Mughal period, yoga continued to be practiced and developed, especially in the courts of the emperors. The Mughal emperors were interested in the physical and spiritual benefits of yoga, and they often invited yogis and spiritual teachers to their courts to teach and practice yoga.

One of the most famous yogis of the Mughal period was Baba Ramdev, who is believed to have lived in the 16th century. Baba Ramdev was a renowned yogi who was said to have developed a series of physical postures that were effective in curing various diseases and promoting health and wellbeing. His teachings were popular among the Mughal emperors, and he was often invited to their courts to teach and demonstrate his yoga postures.

Another important figure in the history of yoga during the Mughal period was Akbar, the third Mughal emperor. Akbar was known for his interest in spirituality and mysticism, and he was particularly interested in the practice of yoga and meditation. Akbar encouraged the development of yoga and meditation in his court, and he invited yogis and spiritual teachers to his court to teach and practice these disciplines.

The Mughal emperors also commissioned the construction of several notable buildings that incorporated elements of yoga and spirituality. One of the most famous of these is the Taj Mahal, a mausoleum built by the emperor Shah Jahan in memory of his wife Mumtaz Mahal. The Taj Mahal is known for its intricate carvings and motifs, many of which are believed to have been inspired by yoga and spiritual symbolism.

Despite the Mughal emperors' patronage of yoga, the practice of yoga continued to be associated with the Hindu and Jain communities in India. Yoga was seen as a way of connecting with the divine and achieving spiritual liberation, and it was often practiced in the context of these religious traditions.

In conclusion, the Mughal Empire was a period of great cultural and artistic development in India, and yoga was an important part of this period. The Mughal emperors were interested in the physical and spiritual benefits of yoga, and they patronized the practice and development of yoga in their courts. The Mughal period also saw the emergence of important yogis and spiritual teachers, such as Baba Ramdev, and the construction of notable buildings, such as the Taj Mahal, that incorporated elements of yoga and spirituality. Despite the Mughal emperors' interest in yoga, the practice continued to be associated with the Hindu and Jain communities in India, and it remained an important aspect of these religious traditions.

The British Raj and the Modernization of Yoga

The British Raj refers to the period of British colonial rule in India from the mid-18th century to the mid-20th century. During this period, the practice of yoga underwent a significant transformation, as it was influenced by Western ideas and practices.

The British colonialists had a complicated relationship with yoga. On the one hand, they saw yoga as a primitive and backward practice that was associated with Hinduism and other indigenous religions. On the other hand, they were interested in the physical and mental benefits of yoga, and they often practiced and promoted yoga in their own communities.

One of the most important figures in the modernization of yoga during the British Raj was Swami Vivekananda. Vivekananda was a Hindu monk who traveled to the United States in the late 19th century to promote Hinduism and yoga. Vivekananda's teachings on yoga emphasized the importance of physical postures, breath control, and meditation, and he helped to popularize these practices in the West.

Another important figure in the modernization of yoga during the British Raj was T. Krishnamacharya. Krishnamacharya was a yoga teacher who developed a style of yoga that emphasized the physical postures, or asanas, and the breath control techniques, or pranayama. Krishnamacharya's style of yoga was influenced by

Western ideas of physical fitness, and it helped to popularize yoga as a form of exercise and stress relief.

During the British Raj, yoga also underwent a process of standardization and codification. This process was led by figures such as B.K.S. Iyengar and Pattabhi Jois, who developed their own styles of yoga that emphasized precise alignment, sequencing, and repetition. These styles of yoga helped to establish a more systematic and scientific approach to yoga, and they helped to make yoga more accessible to a wider audience.

The modernization of yoga during the British Raj also had political implications. As India struggled for independence from British rule, yoga was seen as a symbol of national pride and identity. Yoga was seen as a way of reclaiming India's cultural heritage and asserting its independence from Western influence.

In conclusion, the British Raj had a significant impact on the modernization of yoga in India. The British colonialists were interested in the physical and mental benefits of yoga, and they helped to promote yoga in their own communities. Figures such as Swami Vivekananda and T. Krishnamacharya helped to popularize yoga in the West and develop new styles of yoga that emphasized physical fitness and scientific precision. The modernization of yoga during the British Raj also had political implications, as yoga became a symbol of national pride and identity for India as it struggled for independence from British rule.

Swami Vivekananda and the Introduction of Yoga to the West

Swami Vivekananda was a Hindu monk and spiritual teacher who is widely regarded as one of the most influential figures in the introduction of yoga to the West. Vivekananda was born in 1863 in Calcutta, India, and he spent much of his life traveling the world and promoting Hinduism and yoga.

Vivekananda first gained international recognition at the Parliament of the World's Religions in Chicago in 1893. At the Parliament, Vivekananda delivered a series of lectures on Hinduism and yoga that captivated the audience and established him as a leading authority on these subjects.

Vivekananda's teachings on yoga emphasized the importance of physical postures, breath control, and meditation. He believed that yoga was a practical and scientific method for attaining spiritual liberation and self-realization, and he encouraged his students to approach the practice of yoga with discipline, dedication, and a spirit of inquiry.

Vivekananda's teachings on yoga were highly influential in the West, and they helped to popularize yoga as a spiritual and physical practice. Vivekananda's teachings were also influential in the development of modern yoga, as they emphasized the importance of scientific precision and attention to detail.

One of the most important legacies of Vivekananda's teachings on yoga is the development of the Vedanta

Society, an organization that was founded by Vivekananda and his followers in the United States. The Vedanta Society played an important role in the promotion of Hinduism and yoga in the West, and it helped to establish yoga as a legitimate spiritual practice.

Vivekananda's influence on the development of yoga in the West is still felt today, and his teachings continue to inspire yoga practitioners and spiritual seekers around the world. Vivekananda's emphasis on the practical and scientific aspects of yoga, as well as his focus on discipline and dedication, have helped to establish yoga as a serious and respected practice.

In conclusion, Swami Vivekananda was a key figure in the introduction of yoga to the West. His teachings on yoga emphasized the importance of physical postures, breath control, and meditation, and they helped to popularize yoga as a spiritual and physical practice. Vivekananda's influence on the development of yoga in the West is still felt today, and his teachings continue to inspire yoga practitioners and spiritual seekers around the world. The Vedanta Society, which was founded by Vivekananda and his followers, played an important role in the promotion of Hinduism and yoga in the West, and it helped to establish yoga as a legitimate spiritual practice.

Theosophy and the Influence of Eastern Philosophy on Western Thought

Theosophy is a spiritual and philosophical movement that emerged in the late 19th century and was influential in the development of modern yoga and the introduction of Eastern philosophy to the West. Theosophy was founded by Helena Blavatsky, a Russian spiritual teacher who claimed to have received messages from spiritual beings known as the Masters.

Blavatsky's teachings emphasized the unity of all religions and the importance of spiritual evolution. She drew on a variety of spiritual and philosophical traditions, including Hinduism, Buddhism, and Gnosticism, and she sought to synthesize these traditions into a cohesive spiritual philosophy.

One of the key tenets of Theosophy was the idea of karma, which is a central concept in Hinduism and Buddhism. Theosophy also emphasized the importance of meditation and spiritual practice as a means of achieving spiritual liberation and self-realization.

Theosophy was influential in the development of modern yoga, as it helped to popularize the idea of yoga as a spiritual practice that could be used to achieve spiritual evolution and self-realization. Theosophical teachings on karma, reincarnation, and spiritual evolution also influenced the development of modern yoga philosophy.

The influence of Theosophy on the development of modern yoga is perhaps most evident in the work of the Indian spiritual teacher Jiddu Krishnamurti. Krishnamurti was discovered by Theosophical leaders in India in the early 20th century, and he was promoted as a spiritual leader who would bring about a new era of spiritual awakening. Krishnamurti rejected the Theosophical teachings and established his own teachings on spirituality and meditation, which were heavily influenced by the traditions of Hinduism and Buddhism.

Theosophy also had a broader influence on Western thought, as it helped to introduce Eastern philosophy and spirituality to the West. Theosophical ideas on karma, reincarnation, and spiritual evolution influenced the development of new religious movements and spiritual practices, and they helped to establish a new paradigm for understanding spirituality and the human experience.

In conclusion, Theosophy was a spiritual and philosophical movement that was influential in the development of modern yoga and the introduction of Eastern philosophy to the West. Theosophical teachings on karma, meditation, and spiritual evolution helped to establish yoga as a legitimate spiritual practice, and they influenced the development of modern yoga philosophy. Theosophy also had a broader influence on Western thought, as it helped to introduce Eastern philosophy and spirituality to a wider audience, and it helped to establish a new paradigm for understanding spirituality and the human experience.

The Yoga Renaissance: The 1960s and 70s

The 1960s and 70s were a period of cultural and social upheaval in the West, and they were also a period of renewed interest in yoga and Eastern spirituality. This period is often referred to as the "yoga renaissance," as it saw a surge in the popularity of yoga and the emergence of new forms of yoga practice.

One of the key figures in the yoga renaissance was Swami Satchidananda, an Indian spiritual teacher who founded the Integral Yoga Institute in New York City in 1966. Satchidananda's teachings on yoga emphasized the importance of meditation, self-inquiry, and service to others, and they helped to establish yoga as a tool for personal growth and social transformation.

Another important figure in the yoga renaissance was B.K.S. Iyengar, an Indian yoga teacher who developed a style of yoga that emphasized precise alignment, sequencing, and repetition. Iyengar's style of yoga was influenced by Western ideas of physical fitness and scientific precision, and it helped to make yoga more accessible to a wider audience.

The 1960s and 70s also saw the emergence of new forms of yoga practice, such as Kundalini Yoga, which was developed by Yogi Bhajan, and Jivamukti Yoga, which was developed by David Life and Sharon Gannon. These new forms of yoga practice emphasized the importance of physical postures, breath control, and meditation, and they helped to establish yoga as a dynamic and evolving practice.

The yoga renaissance of the 1960s and 70s was also influenced by broader cultural and social trends, such as the counterculture movement, the civil rights movement, and the feminist movement. Many people saw yoga as a way of challenging the dominant cultural norms and promoting social and political change.

The popularity of yoga during the 1960s and 70s also had a significant impact on the broader culture. Yoga began to appear in popular films, such as "Easy Rider" and "The Graduate," and it was featured in popular magazines, such as "Life" and "Time." Yoga also influenced the development of new forms of music, such as new age and world music.

In conclusion, the yoga renaissance of the 1960s and 70s was a period of renewed interest in yoga and Eastern spirituality. This period saw the emergence of new forms of yoga practice and the development of new styles of yoga teaching. The yoga renaissance was influenced by broader cultural and social trends, and it had a significant impact on the broader culture, influencing the development of music, film, and popular media.

The Beatles and Maharishi Mahesh Yogi

In 1967, the Beatles traveled to India to study Transcendental Meditation with Maharishi Mahesh Yogi, a spiritual teacher from India who had gained international fame as a proponent of meditation and spiritual growth.

The Beatles' interest in meditation was sparked by their growing dissatisfaction with the excesses and pressures of fame, and their desire to find inner peace and spiritual fulfillment. The Beatles were introduced to Maharishi by their manager, Brian Epstein, who had attended one of Maharishi's lectures in London.

The Beatles arrived in India in February 1968 and spent several weeks studying meditation with Maharishi at his ashram in Rishikesh. During their time in India, the Beatles wrote many of the songs that would appear on their "White Album," including "Dear Prudence," "Sexy Sadie," and "Revolution."

The Beatles' association with Maharishi helped to popularize Transcendental Meditation and meditation more generally, and it helped to establish Maharishi as a leading figure in the spiritual and cultural landscape of the 1960s.

However, the Beatles' relationship with Maharishi was not without controversy. Rumors emerged that Maharishi had made inappropriate advances towards one of the female students at the ashram, and the Beatles left India earlier than planned.

The Beatles' time in India had a lasting impact on their music and their personal lives. The songs they wrote during their time in India reflected their growing interest in spirituality and inner peace, and their experiences with meditation helped to shape their outlook on life and their approach to creativity.

The Beatles' association with Maharishi also had a broader impact on the cultural landscape of the 1960s. It helped to popularize meditation and Eastern spirituality in the West, and it paved the way for the emergence of new spiritual and cultural movements in the decades that followed.

In conclusion, the Beatles' association with Maharishi Mahesh Yogi was a significant moment in the history of yoga and Eastern spirituality in the West. The Beatles' interest in meditation helped to popularize Transcendental Meditation and meditation more generally, and it helped to establish Maharishi as a leading figure in the spiritual and cultural landscape of the 1960s. The Beatles' time in India had a lasting impact on their music and their personal lives, and it helped to shape the broader cultural and spiritual movements of the 20th century.

B.K.S. Iyengar and the Development of Iyengar Yoga

B.K.S. Iyengar was an Indian yoga teacher who developed a style of yoga practice that emphasized precise alignment, sequencing, and repetition. Iyengar's approach to yoga was heavily influenced by his own personal struggles with physical limitations and illness, and he developed his style of yoga practice as a way of addressing these challenges.

Iyengar was born in Bellur, India in 1918, and he began practicing yoga at a young age under the guidance of his brother-in-law, the renowned yoga teacher T. Krishnamacharya. Despite his early exposure to yoga, Iyengar struggled with poor health throughout much of his youth, and he suffered from a variety of physical ailments.

In his early twenties, Iyengar began to develop his own approach to yoga practice, which emphasized precise alignment and attention to detail. Iyengar's approach to yoga was influenced by his study of anatomy and physiology, as well as his experiences with physical limitations and illness.

Iyengar's style of yoga practice was also influenced by the broader cultural and social changes of the 20th century. Iyengar's approach to yoga emphasized the importance of physical fitness and scientific precision, and it helped to make yoga more accessible to a wider audience.

Iyengar's approach to yoga became known as Iyengar Yoga, and it is now practiced by millions of people around the world. Iyengar Yoga emphasizes the use of props, such as blocks and straps, to help students achieve correct alignment and deepen their practice. The practice also emphasizes the use of sequencing and repetition to help students build strength, flexibility, and endurance.

Iyengar was a prolific writer and teacher, and he wrote many books on yoga practice and philosophy. His most famous book, "Light on Yoga," is widely regarded as a seminal work in the field of yoga literature, and it has been translated into many languages.

Iyengar continued to teach and practice yoga well into his later years, and he was a leading figure in the world of yoga until his death in 2014 at the age of 95. Iyengar's influence on the world of yoga has been profound, and his legacy continues to shape the practice and teaching of yoga around the world.

In conclusion, B.K.S. Iyengar was an Indian yoga teacher who developed a style of yoga practice that emphasized precise alignment, sequencing, and repetition. Iyengar's approach to yoga was influenced by his own personal struggles with physical limitations and illness, as well as the broader cultural and social changes of the 20th century. Iyengar's style of yoga practice, known as Iyengar Yoga, is now practiced by millions of people around the world, and it has had a profound influence on the practice and teaching of yoga.

Pattabhi Jois and the Ashtanga Vinyasa Yoga System

Pattabhi Jois was an Indian yoga teacher who developed the Ashtanga Vinyasa Yoga system, a style of yoga practice that emphasizes the use of breath-synchronized movements and a specific sequence of postures.

Jois was born in 1915 in a small village in southern India. He began practicing yoga at a young age under the guidance of his teacher, T. Krishnamacharya, and he later went on to develop his own style of yoga practice.

Jois's Ashtanga Vinyasa Yoga system is characterized by a specific sequence of postures, known as the "Primary Series," which is designed to help students develop strength, flexibility, and endurance. The practice also emphasizes the use of breath-synchronized movements, known as "vinyasas," to help students move smoothly between postures and build internal heat.

Jois's Ashtanga Vinyasa Yoga system was heavily influenced by the teachings of T. Krishnamacharya, as well as by the broader cultural and social changes of the 20th century. Jois's approach to yoga emphasized the importance of physical fitness and discipline, and it helped to make yoga more accessible to a wider audience.

Jois began teaching the Ashtanga Vinyasa Yoga system in Mysore, India, in the 1940s, and his students included many prominent figures in the world of yoga, including K.

Pattabhi Jois, who would go on to become a leading figure in the world of yoga in his own right.

Jois continued to teach and develop the Ashtanga Vinyasa Yoga system until his death in 2009 at the age of 93. Today, the Ashtanga Vinyasa Yoga system is practiced by millions of people around the world, and it has had a significant impact on the world of yoga.

In conclusion, Pattabhi Jois was an Indian yoga teacher who developed the Ashtanga Vinyasa Yoga system, a style of yoga practice that emphasizes the use of breath-synchronized movements and a specific sequence of postures. Jois's approach to yoga was influenced by the teachings of T. Krishnamacharya, as well as by the broader cultural and social changes of the 20th century. The Ashtanga Vinyasa Yoga system is now practiced by millions of people around the world, and it has had a significant impact on the world of yoga.

The Evolution of Modern Yoga: Vinyasa and Power Yoga

In recent decades, the world of yoga has undergone a significant evolution, with the emergence of new styles of yoga practice that have challenged and transformed traditional approaches to yoga. Two of the most influential styles of modern yoga practice are Vinyasa Yoga and Power Yoga.

Vinyasa Yoga is a style of yoga practice that emphasizes the use of breath-synchronized movements, known as "vinyasas," to help students move smoothly between postures and build internal heat. Vinyasa Yoga is a dynamic and challenging style of yoga, and it is often characterized by a flowing sequence of postures that can be customized to suit the needs and abilities of individual students.

Power Yoga, on the other hand, is a more intense and athletic style of yoga practice that emphasizes strength, flexibility, and endurance. Power Yoga is often practiced in a heated room and involves a series of dynamic and challenging postures that are designed to push students to their physical limits.

The development of Vinyasa Yoga and Power Yoga is closely tied to the broader cultural and social changes of the late 20th century. These styles of yoga emerged in response to a growing interest in physical fitness and wellness, and they helped to make yoga more accessible and appealing to a wider audience.

Vinyasa Yoga and Power Yoga have had a significant impact on the world of yoga, and they have influenced the development of many other styles of modern yoga practice. These styles of yoga have also helped to broaden the appeal of yoga beyond traditional yoga communities, and they have helped to make yoga a more mainstream and popular form of exercise and wellness practice.

However, the emergence of Vinyasa Yoga and Power Yoga has also been accompanied by some controversy and criticism. Some traditionalists have argued that these styles of yoga place too much emphasis on physical fitness and athleticism, and not enough emphasis on the spiritual and meditative aspects of yoga practice.

In conclusion, Vinyasa Yoga and Power Yoga are two of the most influential styles of modern yoga practice, and they have had a significant impact on the world of yoga. These styles of yoga have helped to make yoga more accessible and appealing to a wider audience, and they have helped to broaden the appeal of yoga beyond traditional yoga communities. However, the emergence of Vinyasa Yoga and Power Yoga has also been accompanied by some controversy and criticism, and they have challenged traditional approaches to yoga practice.

The Rise of Yoga in America: Yoga Journal and Yoga Alliance

The popularity of yoga in America has grown significantly over the past few decades, with millions of people now practicing yoga on a regular basis. Two organizations that have played a significant role in the rise of yoga in America are Yoga Journal and Yoga Alliance.

Yoga Journal is a magazine that was founded in 1975 and is now one of the leading publications on yoga and wellness in the United States. The magazine covers a wide range of topics related to yoga, including practice tips, philosophy, health and wellness, and lifestyle. Yoga Journal has played a significant role in popularizing yoga in America, and it has helped to make yoga more accessible and appealing to a wider audience.

Yoga Alliance is a nonprofit organization that was founded in 1999 with the goal of promoting and supporting the teaching and practice of yoga. The organization sets standards for yoga teacher training programs and certifies yoga teachers who meet those standards. Yoga Alliance has played a significant role in the professionalization of yoga teaching in America, and it has helped to ensure that yoga teachers have the necessary training and qualifications to teach safely and effectively.

The rise of yoga in America is closely tied to the broader cultural and social changes of the late 20th century. The popularity of yoga was fueled by a growing interest in health and wellness, as well as a desire for alternative forms of exercise and spiritual practice. Yoga also appealed to many people as a way to manage stress and improve mental health.

Today, yoga is a thriving industry in America, with millions of people practicing yoga on a regular basis and thousands of yoga studios and teachers across the country. Yoga has become an integral part of the wellness industry, and it is now widely recognized as a legitimate form of exercise and spiritual practice.

However, the rise of yoga in America has also been accompanied by some criticism and controversy. Some traditionalists have argued that the commercialization of yoga has diluted its spiritual and philosophical roots, and that the emphasis on physical fitness and athleticism has detracted from the true essence of yoga practice.

In conclusion, Yoga Journal and Yoga Alliance have played a significant role in the rise of yoga in America, helping to make yoga more accessible and appealing to a wider audience and promoting the professionalization of yoga teaching. The popularity of yoga in America is closely tied to broader cultural and social changes, and it has had a significant impact on the wellness industry. However, the rise of yoga in America has also been accompanied by some controversy and criticism, challenging traditional approaches to yoga practice and raising questions about the commercialization of yoga.

Yoga and the Wellness Industry

Yoga has become a key part of the wellness industry, which encompasses a wide range of products and services related to health, fitness, and self-care. The wellness industry has grown significantly in recent years, with an increasing number of people looking for ways to improve their physical, mental, and emotional health.

Yoga has played a significant role in the growth of the wellness industry, offering a unique and comprehensive approach to health and wellness. The practice of yoga combines physical exercise, meditation, breathwork, and mindfulness, providing a holistic approach to wellness that addresses both the body and the mind.

The popularity of yoga in the wellness industry is closely tied to the broader cultural and social changes of the late 20th century. The 1960s and 70s saw a growing interest in alternative forms of medicine and spiritual practice, and yoga was seen as a way to explore these new ideas and practices.

In the decades since, yoga has become a mainstream form of exercise and wellness practice, with millions of people practicing yoga on a regular basis. Yoga has been shown to have a wide range of health benefits, including improved flexibility, strength, balance, and cardiovascular health. Yoga has also been shown to be effective in managing stress, anxiety, and depression.

The growth of the wellness industry has led to a proliferation of yoga-related products and services, including yoga clothing, mats, props, and accessories, as well as yoga studios, teacher training programs, and retreats. The commercialization of yoga has led to some criticism and controversy, with some traditionalists arguing that the commodification of yoga has detracted from its spiritual and philosophical roots.

Despite these concerns, yoga continues to play a significant role in the wellness industry, and it is likely to continue to grow and evolve in the years to come. Yoga has become an integral part of the wellness industry, offering a unique and holistic approach to health and wellness that addresses both the body and the mind.

In conclusion, yoga has become a key part of the wellness industry, offering a unique and comprehensive approach to health and wellness. The popularity of yoga in the wellness industry is closely tied to the broader cultural and social changes of the late 20th century, and yoga has been shown to have a wide range of health benefits. Despite some criticism and controversy, yoga is likely to continue to play a significant role in the wellness industry, offering a unique and holistic approach to health and wellness that addresses both the body and the mind.

Yoga and the Internet: Yoga in the Digital Age

The rise of the internet and social media has had a significant impact on the world of yoga, transforming the way that people practice and learn about yoga. The internet has made it easier than ever before to access yoga-related content and to connect with other yoga enthusiasts from around the world.

One of the key ways that the internet has impacted yoga is through the proliferation of online yoga classes and tutorials. There are now countless websites and platforms offering online yoga classes, ranging from free resources on YouTube to paid membership sites offering personalized instruction and guidance.

Online yoga classes offer a number of benefits, including convenience, affordability, and accessibility. Online classes allow students to practice yoga from the comfort of their own homes, and they can be accessed at any time, making it easier for people to fit yoga into their busy schedules. Online classes also offer a wider range of styles and teachers than may be available locally, giving students the opportunity to explore different approaches to yoga practice.

Social media has also had a significant impact on the world of yoga, allowing yoga teachers and practitioners to connect with one another and share information and inspiration. Social media platforms like Instagram and Facebook have become popular forums for yoga-related content, with many yoga teachers and influencers using these platforms to share photos and videos of their practice, as well as tips and insights on yoga philosophy and lifestyle.

However, the rise of yoga in the digital age has also raised some concerns and criticisms. Some traditionalists argue that online yoga classes and social media content detract from the true essence of yoga, which is meant to be a deeply personal and transformative practice. Others argue that the commercialization of yoga online has led to a proliferation of unqualified and inexperienced teachers, who may not have the necessary training and qualifications to teach safely and effectively.

Despite these concerns, it is clear that the internet has had a significant impact on the world of yoga, transforming the way that people practice and learn about yoga. Online yoga classes and social media content have made yoga more accessible and appealing to a wider audience, and they have helped to promote the growth and popularity of yoga around the world.

In conclusion, the internet and social media have had a significant impact on the world of yoga, transforming the way that people practice and learn about yoga. Online yoga classes and social media content offer a number of benefits, including convenience, affordability, and accessibility. However, the rise of yoga in the digital age has also raised some concerns and criticisms, challenging traditional approaches to yoga practice and raising questions about the commercialization of yoga online.

Yoga and the Internet: Yoga in the Digital Age

The rise of the internet and social media has had a significant impact on the world of yoga, transforming the way that people practice and learn about yoga. The internet has made it easier than ever before to access yoga-related content and to connect with other yoga enthusiasts from around the world.

One of the key ways that the internet has impacted yoga is through the proliferation of online yoga classes and tutorials. There are now countless websites and platforms offering online yoga classes, ranging from free resources on YouTube to paid membership sites offering personalized instruction and guidance.

Online yoga classes offer a number of benefits, including convenience, affordability, and accessibility. Online classes allow students to practice yoga from the comfort of their own homes, and they can be accessed at any time, making it easier for people to fit yoga into their busy schedules. Online classes also offer a wider range of styles and teachers than may be available locally, giving students the opportunity to explore different approaches to yoga practice.

Social media has also had a significant impact on the world of yoga, allowing yoga teachers and practitioners to connect with one another and share information and inspiration. Social media platforms like Instagram and Facebook have become popular forums for yoga-related content, with many yoga teachers and influencers using these platforms to share photos and videos of their practice, as well as tips and insights on yoga philosophy and lifestyle.

However, the rise of yoga in the digital age has also raised some concerns and criticisms. Some traditionalists argue that online yoga classes and social media content detract from the true essence of yoga, which is meant to be a deeply personal and transformative practice. Others argue that the commercialization of yoga online has led to a proliferation of unqualified and inexperienced teachers, who may not have the necessary training and qualifications to teach safely and effectively.

Despite these concerns, it is clear that the internet has had a significant impact on the world of yoga, transforming the way that people practice and learn about yoga. Online yoga classes and social media content have made yoga more accessible and appealing to a wider audience, and they have helped to promote the growth and popularity of yoga around the world.

In conclusion, the internet and social media have had a significant impact on the world of yoga, transforming the way that people practice and learn about yoga. Online yoga classes and social media content offer a number of benefits, including convenience, affordability, and accessibility. However, the rise of yoga in the digital age has also raised some concerns and criticisms, challenging traditional approaches to yoga practice and raising questions about the commercialization of yoga online.

Yoga and Pop Culture: Yoga in Film and TV

Yoga has become increasingly popular in recent years, and it has also become a fixture of popular culture, with numerous references to yoga appearing in films and television shows. Yoga's presence in pop culture has helped to bring the practice to a wider audience and has helped to demystify some of the misconceptions surrounding yoga.

One of the earliest appearances of yoga in film was in the 1939 film "The Wizard of Oz," in which the Wicked Witch of the West uses a pose called the "Yoga Hatha" to summon a pack of flying monkeys. However, it wasn't until the 1960s and 70s that yoga began to be featured more prominently in film and television.

One of the most iconic depictions of yoga in pop culture is in the 1967 film "You Only Live Twice," in which James Bond is shown practicing yoga as part of his training to become a ninja. This scene helped to establish yoga as a symbol of physical and mental discipline and helped to introduce the practice to a wider audience.

Yoga has also been featured in a number of television shows over the years. One of the most notable examples is the popular 90s sitcom "Friends," in which the character of Ross Geller is a devoted yogi. Ross's passion for yoga helped to popularize the practice among younger audiences and helped to demystify some of the misconceptions surrounding yoga.

In recent years, there has been a surge of interest in yoga in pop culture, with numerous references to yoga appearing in films and television shows. In the 2010 film "Eat Pray Love," the main character, played by Julia Roberts, travels to India to study yoga and meditation. The film helped to popularize the idea of using yoga as a means of personal growth and transformation.

Yoga has also been featured in a number of popular TV shows, including "Orange is the New Black," in which the character of Gloria Mendoza leads a yoga class for the inmates of Litchfield Penitentiary. The show helped to highlight the transformative power of yoga and its ability to bring people together.

Overall, the depiction of yoga in pop culture has helped to bring the practice to a wider audience and has helped to demystify some of the misconceptions surrounding yoga. By portraying yoga as a positive and accessible practice, pop culture has helped to promote the growth and popularity of yoga around the world.

Yoga and Celebrity Culture

Yoga has become increasingly popular among celebrities in recent years, with many famous actors, musicians, and athletes incorporating yoga into their daily routines. The visibility of these high-profile individuals practicing yoga has helped to bring the practice to a wider audience and has helped to promote the growth and popularity of yoga around the world.

One of the earliest celebrity yoga practitioners was actress and fitness guru Jane Fonda, who popularized yoga in the 1980s through her workout videos and books. Fonda's promotion of yoga helped to make the practice more accessible and appealing to a wider audience, and it helped to pave the way for other celebrities to embrace yoga in the decades that followed.

In recent years, a number of high-profile celebrities have become vocal advocates of yoga. One of the most notable examples is actress and entrepreneur Gwyneth Paltrow, who has been an outspoken proponent of yoga and meditation for many years. Paltrow has credited yoga with helping her to manage stress and anxiety and has spoken publicly about the transformative power of the practice.

Other celebrities who practice yoga include actors Jennifer Aniston, Matthew McConaughey, and Robert Downey Jr., as well as musicians like Madonna and Sting. Many of these celebrities have credited yoga with helping them to stay in shape, manage stress, and maintain a sense of balance and perspective in their busy lives.

The popularity of yoga among celebrities has also led to the creation of a number of high-end yoga studios and retreats, catering to the needs and preferences of these high-profile individuals. Many of these studios offer exclusive classes and personalized instruction, allowing celebrities to practice yoga in a more private and personalized setting.

However, the visibility of yoga in celebrity culture has also raised some concerns and criticisms. Some argue that the commercialization of yoga by celebrities and the wellness industry has led to the commodification of the practice, and has detracted from the true essence of yoga, which is meant to be a deeply personal and transformative practice.

Despite these concerns, the popularity of yoga among celebrities has helped to bring the practice to a wider audience and has helped to promote the growth and popularity of yoga around the world. By showcasing the benefits of yoga and making it more accessible and appealing to a wider audience, celebrity culture has helped to demystify some of the misconceptions surrounding yoga and has helped to promote a more inclusive and diverse yoga community.

Yoga in India Today: The Role of the Government

Yoga has always been an integral part of Indian culture, and in recent years, the Indian government has taken steps to promote the practice of yoga both within India and around the world. The government's support for yoga has helped to elevate the practice and to promote its numerous benefits, including its ability to promote physical health, mental well-being, and spiritual growth.

One of the most notable initiatives undertaken by the Indian government in support of yoga is the International Day of Yoga, which was declared by the United Nations in 2014. The initiative, which was proposed by Indian Prime Minister Narendra Modi, aims to raise awareness about the benefits of yoga and to promote the practice around the world. The International Day of Yoga is celebrated annually on June 21, and it has helped to promote the global recognition of yoga as a powerful tool for physical and mental health.

The Indian government has also taken steps to promote the practice of yoga within India, particularly in schools and other educational institutions. In 2016, the Ministry of Human Resource Development issued guidelines for the inclusion of yoga in the school curriculum, with the aim of promoting physical and mental well-being among students. The government has also established the Morarji Desai National Institute of Yoga, which offers training and certification in yoga and related disciplines.

In addition to promoting the practice of yoga, the Indian government has also sought to protect the intellectual property associated with the practice. In 2017, the government granted a trademark to the term "Yoga" under the Trademarks Act, in order to prevent the commercial exploitation of the term by individuals and companies.

Despite the government's support for yoga, there are some concerns that the commercialization of the practice may detract from its true essence and its potential to promote personal and spiritual growth. There are also concerns about the quality and safety of yoga instruction, particularly in the wake of several high-profile cases of injury and even death associated with the practice.

Overall, the Indian government's support for yoga has helped to elevate the practice and to promote its numerous benefits both within India and around the world. By promoting yoga as a powerful tool for physical and mental well-being, the government has helped to bring the practice to a wider audience and to promote its potential for personal and spiritual growth.

Yoga in the West Today: Trends and Developments

Yoga has become increasingly popular in the West in recent years, with millions of people practicing yoga in various forms across the United States, Europe, and other regions. The practice has undergone numerous developments and changes in the West, as it has adapted to local cultures, preferences, and trends. In this chapter, we will explore some of the key trends and developments in the practice of yoga in the West.

1. Mainstream acceptance and integration: Yoga has become increasingly mainstream and integrated into Western culture. Many gyms, health clubs, and wellness centers now offer yoga classes, and many companies have even integrated yoga into their workplace wellness programs. This mainstream acceptance has helped to promote the practice to a wider audience and has helped to dispel some of the misconceptions and stereotypes that have historically been associated with yoga.
2. The rise of different styles and modalities: Yoga has evolved and diversified in the West, with many different styles and modalities emerging in recent years. Some of the most popular styles include Vinyasa, Ashtanga, Hatha, Iyengar, and Bikram yoga, among others. Many practitioners have also adapted the practice to suit their individual needs and preferences, developing hybrid styles and personalized routines.

3. Increased focus on accessibility and inclusivity: There has been a growing emphasis on making yoga accessible and inclusive to people of all ages, abilities, and backgrounds. Many teachers and studios have made efforts to adapt their classes and offerings to accommodate different levels of experience and mobility.
4. The impact of technology: Technology has played a significant role in the evolution of yoga in the West. Many practitioners use online resources and apps to access classes and tutorials, and many teachers use social media to connect with students and promote their offerings. There has also been a rise in virtual and online classes, particularly in the wake of the COVID-19 pandemic, which has forced many studios and teachers to adapt to a more digital format.
5. The commercialization of yoga: The popularity of yoga in the West has led to a significant commercialization of the practice. Many studios, brands, and teachers have developed their own products and offerings, ranging from yoga apparel to retreats and teacher trainings. While this has helped to promote the practice and make it more accessible, it has also raised concerns about the commodification of the practice and the potential for exploitation and appropriation.
6. The role of social and environmental activism: Many practitioners and teachers have sought to connect the practice of yoga with social and environmental activism, promoting values such as mindfulness, compassion, and sustainability. There has been a growing movement towards using yoga as a tool for social change, with many practitioners

and studios donating proceeds to charitable causes and advocating for environmental sustainability.

Overall, the practice of yoga in the West has undergone significant developments and changes in recent years, reflecting the evolving needs and preferences of practitioners and communities. While there are concerns about the commercialization and appropriation of the practice, there is also a growing movement towards making yoga more inclusive, accessible, and socially conscious.

Yoga and Science: The Benefits of Yoga

Yoga has been practiced for thousands of years, and its benefits have been recognized both anecdotally and through scientific research. In recent years, there has been an increasing amount of research on the benefits of yoga, shedding light on the ways in which the practice can improve physical, mental, and emotional well-being. In this chapter, we will explore some of the key benefits of yoga, as supported by scientific research.

1. Improved Physical Health: One of the most well-known benefits of yoga is its ability to improve physical health. Regular practice of yoga has been shown to improve flexibility, balance, strength, and cardiovascular health. A study published in the American Journal of Cardiology found that practicing yoga reduced the risk of heart disease, with participants experiencing improvements in blood pressure, cholesterol levels, and body mass index.
2. Reduced Stress and Anxiety: Yoga is often praised for its ability to promote relaxation and reduce stress and anxiety. This effect has been supported by numerous studies, including a 2016 study published in the Journal of Alternative and Complementary Medicine, which found that practicing yoga reduced symptoms of anxiety and depression in participants.
3. Improved Mental Clarity and Focus: Yoga has been shown to improve mental clarity and focus, as well as cognitive function. A study published in the

Journal of Alzheimer's Disease found that practicing yoga improved memory and cognitive function in older adults, suggesting that it may have potential as a preventative measure against age-related cognitive decline.
4. Improved Sleep: Many people struggle with sleep issues, and yoga has been shown to be an effective tool for improving sleep quality. A study published in the Journal of Clinical Oncology found that practicing yoga improved sleep quality and reduced fatigue in cancer survivors, while a 2015 study published in the Journal of Sleep Disorders and Therapy found that practicing yoga improved sleep quality in people with insomnia.
5. Reduced Inflammation: Chronic inflammation is a known risk factor for a variety of health conditions, including heart disease and cancer. Yoga has been shown to reduce inflammation in the body, with a 2017 study published in the journal Frontiers in Immunology finding that practicing yoga reduced inflammation in breast cancer survivors.
6. Improved Emotional Well-being: Yoga has also been shown to improve emotional well-being, including reducing symptoms of depression and increasing feelings of well-being and contentment. A study published in the journal Evidence-Based Complementary and Alternative Medicine found that practicing yoga improved feelings of self-esteem and reduced symptoms of depression in participants.

Overall, the scientific research on the benefits of yoga is extensive and continues to grow. While the precise mechanisms through which yoga produces these benefits are still being studied, the evidence suggests that the practice has numerous physical, mental, and emotional benefits that can help to improve overall well-being.

Yoga and Social Justice: The Intersection of Yoga and Activism

For many people, yoga is a personal practice that helps them to improve their physical and mental health. However, in recent years, there has been a growing recognition of the potential for yoga to be used as a tool for social justice and activism. In this chapter, we will explore the intersection of yoga and social justice, and the ways in which yoga is being used to promote change in the world.

1. The Roots of Yoga and Social Justice: While yoga has traditionally been seen as a personal practice focused on individual well-being, its roots are deeply intertwined with social justice. The ancient yogic texts emphasize the importance of living a life of service to others, and many of the earliest yogis were social reformers who used yoga as a tool for promoting social change.
2. Yoga and Activism Today: Today, many yoga practitioners are using their practice as a tool for activism and social justice. This can take many forms, from organizing community yoga classes for marginalized communities to using yoga as a tool for self-care and resilience in the face of systemic oppression.
3. Intersectionality and Yog:a One of the key principles of social justice is intersectionality, or the recognition that different forms of oppression are interconnected and cannot be addressed in isolation. In the context of yoga, this means recognizing the ways in which issues like racism, sexism, and classism intersect with the practice of yoga.

4. The Need for Diversity and Inclusion in Yoga: One of the key challenges facing the yoga community today is the lack of diversity and inclusion. Yoga has often been associated with a certain demographic, and many people from marginalized communities have felt excluded from the practice. To address this, there is a growing movement to make yoga more accessible and welcoming to people of all backgrounds.
5. Yoga and Self-Care for Activists: Finally, yoga is increasingly being recognized as a tool for self-care and resilience for activists. The work of promoting social justice can be emotionally and physically demanding, and many activists have turned to yoga as a way to recharge and stay grounded in their work.

Overall, the intersection of yoga and social justice is a rich and complex topic, with many different perspectives and approaches. However, it is clear that there is enormous potential for yoga to be used as a tool for promoting positive change in the world, and many yoga practitioners are working to make this vision a reality. By recognizing the ways in which yoga can intersect with issues of social justice and oppression, we can begin to create a more inclusive and equitable yoga community, and work towards a more just and equitable world.

Conclusion: The Future of Yoga

Yoga has a rich and complex history that has evolved over thousands of years. From its ancient roots in India to its current popularity around the world, yoga has undergone many changes and adaptations. However, as we look to the future of yoga, there are many questions about where the practice is headed. In this final chapter, we will explore some of the key trends and developments shaping the future of yoga.

1. The Growth of Yoga Around the World: One of the most notable trends in the world of yoga is its growing popularity around the world. Yoga is now practiced in countries all over the globe, and there are a growing number of yoga studios, teachers, and practitioners. This growth has been fueled by the increasing recognition of the benefits of yoga, as well as the widespread availability of information about the practice.
2. The Expansion of Yoga Beyond Asana: Another trend that is shaping the future of yoga is the expansion of the practice beyond the physical postures. While asana (the physical postures) is often the entry point for many people into yoga, there is a growing recognition of the importance of the other aspects of yoga, such as pranayama (breathing practices), meditation, and philosophical study. This expansion is leading to a more holistic understanding of yoga, and a deeper exploration of its transformative potential.
3. The Integration of Technology: Another key trend in the future of yoga is the integration of technology. With the increasing use of online

platforms and social media, there are many new opportunities for yoga practitioners to connect with each other and with their teachers. This has led to the growth of online yoga classes and virtual communities, and is changing the way that people approach the practice.
4. The Need for Diversity and Inclusion: As we have seen throughout this book, one of the key challenges facing the yoga community is the lack of diversity and inclusion. In the future of yoga, there is a growing recognition of the need to make the practice more accessible and welcoming to people of all backgrounds. This includes addressing issues such as cultural appropriation, racism, and ableism, and creating spaces that are safe and inclusive for everyone.
5. The Role of Yoga in Society: Finally, the future of yoga will be shaped by its role in society. As we have seen, there is enormous potential for yoga to be used as a tool for social justice and activism, as well as for promoting individual well-being. The future of yoga will depend on how we harness this potential, and on the ways in which we use the practice to address the challenges facing our world.

Overall, the future of yoga is complex and multifaceted, with many different trends and developments shaping the practice. However, one thing is clear: yoga has the potential to continue to evolve and adapt, and to remain a powerful tool for personal and societal transformation. As we look to the future of yoga, it will be important to remain grounded in the principles and values that have guided the practice throughout its long and storied history, while also remaining open to new possibilities and opportunities for growth and evolution.

Thank you for taking the time to read this book on the history of yoga. We hope that it has provided you with a deeper understanding of this ancient practice and its evolution throughout history.

If you enjoyed this book, we would greatly appreciate it if you could take a few moments to leave a positive review. Your feedback is incredibly valuable and will help others to discover and benefit from this book as well.

Once again, thank you for your interest in yoga and for choosing to read this book. We wish you all the best on your yoga journey, and hope that the practice continues to bring you joy, peace, and transformation.

Printed in Great Britain
by Amazon